UNLOCKING LYMPHOCYTIC COLITIS

A Comprehensive Guide to
Diagnosis, Treatment, and Living
Well with Chronic Bowel
Inflammation

Adams .U. Morris

Copyright © [2023] by [Adams .U .Morris]

All rights reserved.

Publish by Adams .U. Morris

Disclaimer: the opinion and views expressed in this book are those of the author and do not necessarily reflect the policy or position of any character or organization mention in this book

TABLE OF CONTENTS

CHAPTER 1

Introduction to Lymphocytic Colitis

In this opening chapter, we delve into the world of lymphocytic colitis, a condition that affects many people but is often not widely understood. We will start by discussing what lymphocytic colitis is, its prevalence, who is most commonly affected, and why it's crucial for both patients and healthcare providers to grasp the intricacies of this condition.

What is Lymphocytic Colitis?

Lymphocytic colitis, often referred to as LC, is a type of inflammatory bowel disease (IBD) that primarily affects the colon or large intestine. It's characterized by chronic inflammation in the colon's lining, leading to various gastrointestinal symptoms. LC is considered a subtype of microscopic colitis, which also includes collagenous colitis.

The Prevalence of Lymphocytic Colitis

Lymphocytic colitis might not be as widely recognized as other gastrointestinal conditions like Crohn's disease or ulcerative colitis, but it's more common than you might think. While the exact prevalence can vary from region to region, studies have shown that it affects primarily adults, with a peak onset typically occurring in people between the ages of 50 and 60.

Who is Most Commonly Affected?

Lymphocytic colitis does not discriminate when it comes to gender; both men and women are susceptible. However, it tends to occur more frequently in women. Additionally, individuals with certain risk factors, such as a family history of IBD or autoimmune diseases like celiac disease, might have a higher likelihood of developing LC.

The Importance of Understanding Lymphocytic Colitis

Why is it essential for both patients and healthcare providers to understand lymphocytic colitis? The answer lies in the potential for misdiagnosis and the impact this condition can have on an individual's quality of life.

Misdiagnosis can be a significant issue because the symptoms of LC can mimic those of other gastrointestinal disorders, such as irritable bowel syndrome (IBS). Without a proper diagnosis, patients might not receive the appropriate treatment, leading to ongoing discomfort and uncertainty.

Furthermore, the chronic nature of lymphocytic colitis can significantly affect a person's daily life. Symptoms like chronic diarrhea, abdominal pain, and weight loss can be physically and emotionally draining. Therefore, understanding the condition and its management options can empower patients to take control of their health and improve their overall well-being.

For healthcare providers, recognizing the symptoms and characteristics of lymphocytic colitis is crucial for accurate diagnosis and treatment. Awareness of this condition enables doctors to consider LC as a potential diagnosis, particularly in patients with persistent gastrointestinal issues. Early diagnosis and appropriate management can lead to better outcomes and an improved quality of life for patients.

In the following chapters, we will delve deeper into the intricacies of lymphocytic colitis, exploring the anatomy and function of the lymphatic system, the signs and symptoms of the condition, potential causes and risk factors, and various treatment options, both medical and lifestyle-based. We will also hear from patients who have firsthand experience living with lymphocytic colitis, as well as experts in the field who can provide insights into the latest research and future directions for understanding and managing this condition.

As we continue this journey of exploration, it's important to remember that lymphocytic colitis is a real and impactful condition that affects individuals and their families. By gaining a deeper understanding of LC, we can work together to improve diagnosis, treatment, and support systems for those living with this often-overlooked form of inflammatory bowel disease.

CHAPTER 2

Understanding the Anatomy and Function of the Lymphatic System

In this chapter, we embark on a journey to unravel the complexities of the lymphatic system. Understanding this intricate network is crucial for comprehending how it relates to lymphocytic colitis, a condition discussed in this book. We'll explore the lymphatic system's anatomy, its vital functions, and its interactions with the gastrointestinal tract.

The Lymphatic System Unveiled

The lymphatic system is often overshadowed by its more famous counterpart, the circulatory system, which includes the heart and blood vessels. However, this system is no less important. It plays a critical role in maintaining overall health and well-being.

At its core, the lymphatic system is a network of vessels, nodes, and organs that work together to transport lymph, a clear fluid that contains white blood cells (lymphocytes), throughout the body. The lymphatic system is distributed throughout the body, much like blood vessels. It's a comprehensive network that reaches almost every tissue and organ.

The Lymphatic System's Crucial Functions

Now, let's explore why the lymphatic system is indispensable for our health:

1. **Immune Defense:** One of the primary functions of the lymphatic system is to

support the body's immune defenses. Lymphocytes, including B cells and T cells, are essential components of our immune system. They are produced in bone marrow and mature in the lymphatic tissues, such as the thymus gland and lymph nodes. Once matured, these lymphocytes play a vital role in recognizing and combating infections and foreign invaders.

2. **Fluid Balance:** The lymphatic system helps maintain fluid balance in the body. It collects excess fluid

from body tissues, preventing swelling (edema). This fluid is then transported back into the bloodstream via the lymphatic vessels.

3. **Absorption of Nutrients:** Within the gastrointestinal tract, the lymphatic system plays a critical role in the absorption of dietary fats. Specialized lymphatic vessels called lacteals absorb dietary fats and fat-soluble vitamins from the intestines and transport them to the bloodstream.

The Lymphatic System and the Gastrointestinal Tract

Now that we have a basic understanding of the lymphatic system's functions, let's explore its connection to the gastrointestinal tract and its relevance to lymphocytic colitis:

Lymphatic Vessels in the GI Tract: The gastrointestinal tract is rich in lymphatic vessels. These vessels are responsible for absorbing nutrients from digested food and transporting them throughout the body. In particular, the small intestine contains numerous lacteals, specialized lymphatic vessels that absorb dietary fats and fat-soluble vitamins.

Lymphatic System and Lymphocytic Colitis: Lymphocytic colitis primarily affects the colon, which is part of the digestive system. While the exact cause of lymphocytic colitis remains unclear, there is evidence to suggest that the lymphatic system might play a role in the development of this condition.

In lymphocytic colitis, the immune system appears to be overactive in the colon's lining. Lymphocytes, a type of white blood cell found in the lymphatic system, are often present in higher numbers in the colonic tissue of individuals with this condition. This immune response leads to chronic inflammation and the symptoms associated with lymphocytic colitis, such as chronic diarrhea and abdominal pain.

While the exact relationship between the lymphatic system and lymphocytic colitis is still being studied, it's believed that immune cells, including lymphocytes, might play a role in the inflammation seen in the colon of affected individuals.

Understanding this connection is crucial for developing targeted treatments and therapies for lymphocytic colitis.

The Link Between Lymphatic Health and Lymphocytic Colitis

Maintaining a healthy lymphatic system is essential for overall well-being. While lymphocytic colitis is primarily a condition of the colon, the health of the entire lymphatic system can influence how the body responds to inflammation and infection.

Proper nutrition, regular exercise, and stress management are factors that can positively impact lymphatic health. For example, maintaining a balanced diet with essential nutrients supports the production of lymphocytes and other immune cells, while physical activity can help promote the circulation of lymphatic fluid throughout the body.

In individuals with lymphocytic colitis, lifestyle choices that support overall health can complement medical treatments and improve their quality of life. Additionally, research into the interaction between the lymphatic system and this condition may lead to more targeted therapies in the future.

In the upcoming chapters of this book, we will delve deeper into the signs, symptoms, and diagnosis of lymphocytic colitis, exploring the challenges patients face in obtaining an accurate diagnosis and the various medical and lifestyle-based treatment options available. We will also examine potential causes and risk factors associated with this condition, shedding light on the factors that might contribute to its development.

By the end of this book, you'll have a comprehensive understanding of lymphocytic colitis, from its impact on patients' lives to the latest research efforts aimed at improving our understanding and management of this complex condition.

CHAPTER 3

Signs, Symptoms, and Diagnosis of Lymphocytic Colitis

In this chapter, we dive into the often puzzling and sometimes elusive signs, symptoms, and diagnosis of lymphocytic colitis. Understanding these aspects is critical as it forms the foundation for identifying and managing this condition effectively.

The Enigmatic Nature of Lymphocytic Colitis Symptoms

Lymphocytic colitis is known for its enigmatic and diverse range of symptoms, which can make it challenging to diagnose. These symptoms often overlap with other gastrointestinal disorders, such as irritable bowel syndrome (IBS) or even other forms of inflammatory bowel disease (IBD), like Crohn's disease or ulcerative colitis. This complexity underscores the importance of accurate diagnosis.

Common Symptoms of Lymphocytic Colitis:

1. **Chronic Diarrhea:** The hallmark symptom of

lymphocytic colitis is chronic, watery diarrhea. Individuals may experience frequent bowel movements, often multiple times a day, which can be socially and physically disruptive.

2. **Abdominal Pain:** Many people with lymphocytic colitis report abdominal discomfort or cramping, which can range from mild to severe.

3. **Weight Loss:** Prolonged diarrhea and malabsorption of nutrients can lead to weight loss, which can be concerning for patients.

4. **Dehydration:** Chronic diarrhea can cause dehydration, leading to symptoms like excessive thirst, dry mouth, and fatigue.

5. **Bloating and Gas:** Some individuals experience bloating and increased gas production.

6. **Urgency:** A frequent urge to have a bowel movement, often with little warning, is common.

The Diagnostic Challenge

The symptoms of lymphocytic colitis can be distressing and

persistent, often prompting individuals to seek medical attention. However, diagnosing lymphocytic colitis is not always straightforward. Here's why:

1. **Overlapping Symptoms:** As mentioned earlier, the symptoms of lymphocytic colitis can overlap with several other gastrointestinal conditions. This overlap can lead to misdiagnosis or delayed diagnosis.

2. **Invisible to Imaging:** Standard imaging tests like X-rays or CT scans may not reveal the inflammation in

the colon lining seen in lymphocytic colitis. Unlike some other forms of IBD, such as Crohn's disease, which can involve visible structural changes, lymphocytic colitis primarily affects the microscopic appearance of the colon lining.

3. **Biopsy Requirement:** To definitively diagnose lymphocytic colitis, a biopsy of the colon lining is usually necessary. During a colonoscopy or sigmoidoscopy, small tissue samples are taken from the

colon for examination under a microscope. In lymphocytic colitis, these biopsies reveal characteristic changes, including an increased number of lymphocytes in the colon's epithelial lining.

The Diagnostic Process

The diagnostic process for lymphocytic colitis typically involves several steps:

1. **Medical History and Symptoms:** The process often begins with a thorough medical history and

discussion of the patient's symptoms. This helps the healthcare provider rule out other potential causes of gastrointestinal symptoms.

2. **Physical Examination:** A physical examination may be performed to check for signs of abdominal tenderness or other abnormalities.

3. **Blood Tests:** Blood tests may be conducted to rule out other conditions and assess for markers of inflammation.

4. **Imaging Tests:** While imaging tests may not reveal specific changes related to lymphocytic colitis, they can

help rule out other conditions or complications.

5. **Colonoscopy or Sigmoidoscopy:** These procedures involve the insertion of a flexible tube with a camera into the colon. Biopsies are taken during these procedures to examine the colon lining.

6. **Histopathology:** The biopsied tissue samples are sent to a pathology laboratory, where they are examined under a microscope. The presence of increased lymphocytes in the

colon lining is a key finding in lymphocytic colitis.

The Importance of an Accurate Diagnosis

Accurate diagnosis of lymphocytic colitis is essential for several reasons:

1. **Appropriate Treatment:** An accurate diagnosis allows healthcare providers to prescribe treatments specifically tailored to lymphocytic colitis. This can help manage symptoms and improve the patient's quality of life.

2. **Avoiding Unnecessary Medications:** Misdiagnosis can lead to unnecessary treatments and medications, which may not effectively address the underlying condition.

3. **Quality of Life:** Chronic diarrhea and other symptoms of lymphocytic colitis can significantly impact a person's quality of life. An accurate diagnosis can provide clarity and guidance for managing these symptoms.

4. **Monitoring and Management:** An accurate

diagnosis enables healthcare providers to monitor the condition's progression and adjust treatment as needed.

Challenges in Diagnosis and Advocacy

For many individuals, the road to a lymphocytic colitis diagnosis can be long and frustrating. They may encounter misdiagnoses or dismissive attitudes from healthcare providers. This highlights the importance of advocacy and self-advocacy within the medical system. Patients should feel empowered to seek second opinions and advocate for the tests and evaluations necessary to reach an accurate diagnosis.

In the next chapter, we will explore potential causes and risk factors associated with lymphocytic colitis, shedding light on the factors that might contribute to the development of this condition. Understanding these aspects can further enhance our grasp of lymphocytic colitis and pave the way for more effective management and treatment strategies.

CHAPTER 4

Potential Causes and Risk Factors of Lymphocytic Colitis

In this chapter, we delve into the intriguing question of what might cause lymphocytic colitis and the risk factors that make some individuals more susceptible to this condition than others. Understanding the potential triggers and contributors is essential for shedding light on the development of lymphocytic colitis.

The Mystery of Lymphocytic Colitis Causes

Lymphocytic colitis is considered an idiopathic condition, which means its exact cause remains unknown. However, researchers have identified several factors that may contribute to its development. It's essential to remember that lymphocytic colitis is a complex disorder, and its causes are likely multifactorial.

Autoimmune Factors:

1. **Immune System Dysfunction:** Lymphocytic colitis is categorized as an

autoimmune disorder. In autoimmune conditions, the immune system, which is supposed to protect the body, mistakenly attacks healthy tissues. In lymphocytic colitis, immune cells, specifically lymphocytes, accumulate in the colon's lining, leading to chronic inflammation.

2. **Association with Other Autoimmune Diseases:** Some individuals with lymphocytic colitis also have other autoimmune diseases, such as celiac disease, rheumatoid arthritis, or

thyroid disorders. This suggests a potential link between autoimmune factors and lymphocytic colitis.

Genetic Factors:

1. **Family History:** There is evidence to suggest that genetic factors may play a role in the development of lymphocytic colitis. Some individuals with lymphocytic colitis have a family history of autoimmune conditions or gastrointestinal disorders, indicating a potential genetic predisposition.

2. **Genetic Variants:** Research is ongoing to identify specific genetic variants that may increase the risk of lymphocytic colitis. Identifying these variants could provide valuable insights into the condition's underlying mechanisms.

Environmental Factors:

1. **Infections:** Some researchers have explored the possibility that viral or bacterial infections may trigger lymphocytic colitis in susceptible individuals.

However, no specific infectious agent has been consistently linked to the condition.

2. **Dietary Factors:** While not a direct cause, dietary factors may influence the development or exacerbation of lymphocytic colitis. Some individuals find that certain foods, such as spicy or high-fat foods, worsen their symptoms. Additionally, if someone with undiagnosed celiac disease consumes gluten, it can lead to similar symptoms as lymphocytic colitis.

Medications and Triggers:

1. **Medications:** Some medications have been associated with the development of lymphocytic colitis. These include nonsteroidal anti-inflammatory drugs (NSAIDs), such as ibuprofen, and proton pump inhibitors (PPIs), which are used to treat acid reflux. It's essential for individuals taking these medications to be aware of potential side effects and discuss any

concerns with their healthcare provider.

2. **Stress:** While not a direct cause, stress can exacerbate symptoms of lymphocytic colitis and other gastrointestinal conditions. Stress management techniques may be helpful for individuals with this condition.

Hormonal Factors:

1. **Gender:** Lymphocytic colitis appears to affect women more frequently than men. This gender disparity suggests that hormonal

factors may contribute to the condition's development. Hormonal fluctuations during menopause, for example, might play a role in symptom onset or severity.

Understanding Risk Factors

While we have discussed potential causes and contributing factors, it's important to note that having one or more of these risk factors does not guarantee the development of lymphocytic colitis. Many individuals with the condition do not have identifiable risk factors, further highlighting its complexity.

The Role of Diagnosis in Understanding Causes and Risk Factors

Diagnosing lymphocytic colitis is a crucial step in understanding its causes and risk factors. Through careful evaluation and analysis of patient data, researchers can identify patterns and associations that may shed light on the condition's origins.

Ongoing Research and Future Directions

Research into the causes and risk factors of lymphocytic colitis is ongoing. Scientists are working to uncover the specific genetic and environmental triggers that may increase an individual's susceptibility to this condition. Additionally, investigations into the role of the immune system and its interactions with the colon are advancing our understanding of lymphocytic colitis.

Personalized Approaches to Treatment and Prevention

As our understanding of lymphocytic colitis causes and risk factors evolves, it has the potential to lead to more personalized approaches to treatment and prevention. For example, identifying specific genetic markers associated with the condition could allow for targeted therapies that address the underlying mechanisms of lymphocytic colitis.

Patient Advocacy and Support

Living with lymphocytic colitis can be challenging, especially for those facing the uncertainty of its causes and risk factors. Patient advocacy and support networks play a crucial role in providing information, resources, and a sense of community for individuals and their families dealing with this condition.

Conclusion

Lymphocytic colitis remains a condition with many unanswered questions about its causes and risk factors. While it is known to have autoimmune and genetic components, the interplay of these factors with environmental triggers is still a subject of ongoing research. Understanding these aspects is not only essential for unraveling the mysteries of lymphocytic colitis but also for developing more effective strategies for its management and prevention.

In the following chapters, we will explore treatment options for lymphocytic colitis, both medical and lifestyle-based, and provide insights into how individuals can manage their symptoms and improve their quality of life. We will also delve into the personal experiences of patients who have learned to navigate the challenges of living with lymphocytic colitis and the role of patient advocacy in raising awareness and supporting those affected by this condition.

CHAPTER 5

Treatment Options for Lymphocytic Colitis

In this chapter, we'll explore the various treatment options available for lymphocytic colitis. Effective management of this condition is essential to alleviate symptoms, improve quality of life, and minimize its impact on daily activities. Treatment strategies for lymphocytic colitis encompass both medical interventions and lifestyle modifications.

Medical Treatment Options

1. **Anti-Diarrheal Medications:** Chronic diarrhea is a hallmark symptom of lymphocytic colitis. Anti-diarrheal medications like loperamide (Imodium) can help reduce the frequency and urgency of bowel movements. These medications work by slowing down the movement of stool through the intestines.

2. **Budesonide (Corticosteroid):** Budesonide is a corticosteroid medication that can be used to manage the inflammation associated

with lymphocytic colitis. Unlike traditional corticosteroids, budesonide has fewer systemic side effects because it is designed to release its active ingredient specifically in the colon. This targeted approach can help reduce inflammation without affecting the entire body.

3. **Immunosuppressive Medications:** In some cases, immunosuppressive medications, such as azathioprine or mercaptopurine, may be prescribed to suppress the

overactive immune response seen in lymphocytic colitis. These medications are typically used when other treatments have not provided sufficient relief or in cases of severe disease.

4. **Anti-TNF Therapy:** Tumor necrosis factor (TNF) is a protein involved in inflammation. Anti-TNF therapies, like infliximab or adalimumab, are used in certain autoimmune conditions to reduce inflammation by targeting TNF. These medications are sometimes considered for

individuals with lymphocytic colitis who do not respond to other treatments.

Lifestyle-Based Treatment Options

1. **Dietary Modifications:** Making dietary adjustments can significantly impact the management of lymphocytic colitis. While there is no one-size-fits-all diet for this condition, some dietary modifications may help reduce symptoms. These include:

   - **Low-Fat Diet:** Reducing dietary fat

intake can help alleviate diarrhea in some individuals.

- **Low-Fiber Diet:** A low-fiber diet may be recommended during active flare-ups to minimize irritation of the colon.

- **Avoidance of Trigger Foods:** Identifying and avoiding foods that exacerbate symptoms is crucial. Common triggers include caffeine, alcohol, spicy foods, and artificial sweeteners.

- o **Lactose Avoidance:** Some individuals with lymphocytic colitis may also have lactose intolerance. Avoiding dairy products or using lactase supplements can be helpful.

2. **Hydration:** Chronic diarrhea can lead to dehydration. Staying well-hydrated is essential. Oral rehydration solutions or electrolyte-rich drinks can be beneficial.

3. **Stress Management:** Stress can exacerbate gastrointestinal symptoms. Practicing stress management techniques such as deep breathing, meditation, or yoga can help reduce stress-related flares.

The Importance of Individualized Treatment

Lymphocytic colitis is a highly individualized condition, and what works for one person may not work for another. Therefore, treatment plans must be tailored to the specific needs and symptoms of each patient. A gastroenterologist or healthcare provider experienced in managing inflammatory bowel diseases like lymphocytic colitis can work closely with patients to develop personalized treatment strategies.

Monitoring and Follow-Up

Regular monitoring and follow-up appointments are essential to assess the effectiveness of treatment and make any necessary adjustments. Patients should communicate openly with their healthcare providers about their symptoms and any changes in their condition. These appointments also provide an opportunity to address any concerns or side effects of medications.

The Role of Patient Education

Empowering patients with knowledge about lymphocytic colitis and its treatment options is crucial. When patients understand their condition and treatment plan, they are better equipped to make informed decisions about their health and advocate for their needs.

The Challenge of Flare-Ups and Remission

Lymphocytic colitis can have a relapsing-remitting course, meaning that symptoms may come and go over time. Understanding the nature of flare-ups and remission is essential for patients and their healthcare providers.

During a flare-up, symptoms may worsen or return after a period of remission. This can be frustrating, but it's important to remember that flare-ups do not necessarily indicate treatment failure. They are a natural part of the disease process. Adjusting treatment as needed during flare-ups can help bring symptoms under control.

Conversely, during periods of remission, symptoms may improve or disappear entirely. However, it's essential for individuals with lymphocytic colitis to continue their treatment plan and follow-up care even when they are feeling well. This proactive approach can help maintain symptom control and reduce the risk of future flare-ups.

Long-Term Outlook and Quality of Life

Lymphocytic colitis is typically a chronic condition, meaning it persists over time. However, with appropriate treatment and lifestyle modifications, many individuals with lymphocytic colitis are able to manage their symptoms effectively and maintain a good quality of life.

It's important to acknowledge that living with lymphocytic colitis can present challenges, both physical and emotional. The chronic nature of the condition and its impact on daily life can be distressing. This is where the support of healthcare providers, patient advocacy groups, and peer support networks becomes invaluable.

Patient Perspectives and Shared Experiences

In the next chapter of this book, we will hear from individuals who have been diagnosed with lymphocytic colitis. They will share their personal experiences, challenges, and strategies for managing this condition. These stories offer valuable insights and inspiration for others living with lymphocytic colitis, as well as their caregivers and loved ones.

In conclusion, while lymphocytic colitis may present complex challenges, it is a condition that can be managed with the right approach. Treatment options, both medical and lifestyle-based, provide hope for symptom relief and an improved quality of life for individuals living with this condition.

CHAPTER 6

Living with Lymphocytic Colitis: Coping Strategies

In this chapter, we will explore the daily challenges faced by individuals living with lymphocytic colitis and provide coping strategies to help them navigate life with this condition. Chronic illnesses can have a significant impact on a person's physical and emotional well-being, and learning how to cope effectively is crucial for maintaining the best possible quality of life.

Understanding the Daily Impact

Living with lymphocytic colitis can be challenging due to the persistent symptoms and uncertainty about when flare-ups might occur. The condition's primary symptom, chronic diarrhea, can be particularly disruptive to daily life. Individuals may face:

1. **Social Limitations:** Fear of not being near a bathroom can lead to social isolation

and avoidance of activities or events.

2. **Work Challenges:** Frequent restroom breaks and unpredictable symptoms can interfere with work responsibilities.

3. **Emotional Impact:** Dealing with chronic symptoms can lead to frustration, anxiety, and depression.

4. **Nutritional Concerns:** Managing dietary restrictions and potential weight loss can be daunting.

Coping Strategies for Daily Life

1. **Open Communication:** Talk to your healthcare provider about your symptoms and concerns. They can adjust your treatment plan or suggest alternative therapies as needed. Don't hesitate to ask questions and seek clarification about your condition.

2. **Dietary Management:** Keep a food diary to identify trigger foods that worsen your symptoms. A registered

dietitian can help you create a personalized diet plan that minimizes discomfort while meeting your nutritional needs.

3. **Hydration:** Chronic diarrhea can lead to dehydration. Stay hydrated by sipping water throughout the day and considering oral rehydration solutions.

4. **Stress Reduction:** Explore stress-reduction techniques like meditation, deep breathing exercises, or yoga. Reducing stress can help minimize the impact of

emotional triggers on your symptoms.

5. **Travel Planning:** If you love to travel, plan trips with proximity to restroom facilities in mind. Also, bring any necessary medications or supplies with you.

6. **Workplace Accommodations:** If necessary, discuss workplace accommodations with your employer. These may include flexible work hours or access to a restroom when needed.

Support Networks and Online Communities

Navigating lymphocytic colitis can be less daunting when you connect with others who share similar experiences. Support networks and online communities can provide a sense of belonging and a wealth of information. Here's how they can help:

1. **Emotional Support:** Sharing your feelings and experiences with others who understand what you're going through can be immensely comforting.

You're not alone in this journey.

2. **Practical Advice:** Fellow patients may offer practical tips and advice for managing daily life with lymphocytic colitis, from dietary suggestions to travel hacks.

3. **Advocacy:** Being part of a community can empower you to advocate for yourself and others. You can raise awareness about lymphocytic colitis and share your experiences with healthcare providers, researchers, and policymakers.

4. **Knowledge Sharing:** Online communities are a valuable source of information about the latest research, treatments, and developments related to lymphocytic colitis.

5. **Peer Support:** Hearing stories of resilience and success from individuals who have lived with lymphocytic colitis for years can provide hope and inspiration.

Patient Stories: Personal Experiences

To gain a deeper understanding of what it's like to live with lymphocytic colitis and the coping strategies that individuals employ, we'll now hear from people who have been diagnosed with the condition. These personal stories offer a glimpse into the challenges they've faced and the ways they've learned to manage lymphocytic colitis.

Story 1: Sarah's Journey

Sarah was diagnosed with lymphocytic colitis in her early 40s. She recalls the initial frustration of experiencing chronic diarrhea without a clear diagnosis.

"I felt like I was living in the bathroom, and it was taking a toll on my mental health," she says.

Coping Strategy: Sarah found solace in a support group for individuals with gastrointestinal conditions. Through shared experiences, she learned about dietary modifications that helped control her symptoms. "I never realized how much food could impact my condition until I started hearing what worked for others," she explains.

Story 2: Mark's Experience

Mark was diagnosed with lymphocytic colitis in his late 50s, following a prolonged period of unexplained diarrhea. "It was challenging because I was nearing retirement, and I didn't want my symptoms to dictate my life," he says.

Coping Strategy: Mark worked closely with his gastroenterologist to find a medication that provided relief. He also embraced stress-reduction techniques like mindfulness meditation, which helped him manage symptoms during stressful periods. "Mindfulness gave me a sense of control over my body and my condition," he shares.

Story 3: Emily's Support System

Emily, a college student, was diagnosed with lymphocytic colitis at a young age. She found herself dealing with the challenges of managing her condition while pursuing higher education.

Coping Strategy: Emily sought support from her college's disability services office. They provided accommodations like priority restroom access and flexibility with deadlines during flare-ups. "Having that support in place made it possible for me to focus on my studies without constantly worrying about my symptoms," she says.

The Power of Resilience

These personal stories highlight the resilience of individuals living with lymphocytic colitis. While the condition can present significant challenges, it doesn't define their lives. Through a combination of medical treatment, lifestyle adjustments, and support networks, many people find ways to manage their symptoms effectively and maintain a fulfilling life.

In the next chapter, we will explore the latest research and future directions in the field of lymphocytic colitis. Advancements in understanding this condition are ongoing, and these developments offer hope for improved treatments and a deeper understanding of its causes and mechanisms.

CHAPTER 7

The Future of Lymphocytic Colitis: Research and Advancements

In this chapter, we'll delve into the exciting world of research and advancements in the field of lymphocytic colitis. Understanding where the scientific community is heading can provide hope for improved treatments, a better understanding of the condition's causes, and enhanced support for individuals living with lymphocytic colitis.

Challenges in Lymphocytic Colitis Research

Lymphocytic colitis has historically been a relatively understudied condition compared to other gastrointestinal disorders like Crohn's disease or ulcerative colitis. Several factors have contributed to these challenges:

1. **Low Awareness:** Limited awareness of lymphocytic colitis among the general public and even some healthcare providers has led

to underdiagnosis and underreporting of cases.

2. **Heterogeneity:** Lymphocytic colitis is a heterogeneous condition, meaning it can present differently from person to person. This variability makes it challenging to conduct large-scale studies and draw definitive conclusions.

3. **Lack of Biomarkers:** Unlike some other diseases, lymphocytic colitis lacks specific biomarkers that can be easily detected in blood

tests or other diagnostic methods.

Despite these challenges, researchers and healthcare professionals are increasingly recognizing the importance of studying lymphocytic colitis, and significant progress has been made in recent years.

Current Areas of Research

1. **Genetic Factors:** Scientists are investigating the genetic underpinnings of lymphocytic colitis. Identifying specific genetic markers associated with the

condition could lead to more targeted treatments and a better understanding of its causes.

2. **Immune System Function:** Research is focused on understanding how the immune system interacts with the colon in individuals with lymphocytic colitis. This knowledge could pave the way for immune-modulating therapies.

3. **Microbiome Studies:** The gut microbiome, the community of microorganisms in the digestive tract, plays a

crucial role in gastrointestinal health. Researchers are exploring whether imbalances in the gut microbiome contribute to the development or exacerbation of lymphocytic colitis.

4. **Biomarker Discovery:** Efforts are underway to identify specific biomarkers associated with lymphocytic colitis. These biomarkers could simplify diagnosis and monitoring of the condition.

5. **Treatment Advancements:** Clinical trials and research studies

are evaluating the effectiveness of new medications and therapies for lymphocytic colitis. This includes testing novel anti-inflammatory drugs and immune-modulating treatments.

Patient Involvement in Research

Patient involvement in research is gaining recognition as a valuable and essential component of advancing our understanding of lymphocytic colitis. Here's how patients can contribute:

1. **Participating in Clinical Trials:** Clinical trials are essential for testing new treatments and therapies. Patients can consider participating in trials if they meet the eligibility criteria.

2. **Sharing Experiences:** Patients can share their experiences with researchers and healthcare providers. These insights can help shape research priorities and improve the patient experience.

3. **Advocacy:** Patient advocacy groups play a critical role in raising

awareness about lymphocytic colitis and advocating for increased research funding and support.

The Promise of Personalized Medicine

As research in lymphocytic colitis advances, there is increasing hope for personalized medicine approaches. Personalized medicine takes into account an individual's unique genetic makeup, lifestyle, and other factors to tailor treatment plans specifically to their needs. In the future, individuals with lymphocytic colitis may benefit from therapies that are precisely matched to their condition.

Supporting Patients Through Research

For individuals living with lymphocytic colitis, the advancements in research bring hope for better treatment options and a deeper understanding of their condition. It's important for patients to stay informed about ongoing research and to consider participating in studies if they are eligible and interested.

Advocacy and Awareness

Raising awareness about lymphocytic colitis is essential for driving research efforts and improving support for affected individuals. Advocacy groups and individuals can play a crucial role in this regard:

1. **Education:** Educating the public, healthcare providers, and policymakers about lymphocytic colitis is fundamental to increasing awareness.

2. **Funding:** Advocacy efforts can help secure funding for research into lymphocytic colitis, which is often

underfunded compared to other gastrointestinal conditions.

3. **Support Networks:** Advocacy groups provide a platform for individuals and their families to connect, share experiences, and advocate for better care and support.

A Brighter Future for Lymphocytic Colitis

While lymphocytic colitis can present significant challenges, the future holds promise for improved diagnosis, treatment, and support for individuals living with this condition. Advances in genetics, immunology, and microbiome research are providing new insights into the condition's mechanisms and potential therapeutic targets.

As researchers continue to unravel the mysteries of lymphocytic colitis, individuals with the condition can look forward to more personalized and effective treatment options. Patient advocacy and involvement in research will remain vital in driving progress and improving the lives of those affected by lymphocytic colitis.

Conclusion

In this chapter, we've explored the exciting world of research and advancements in the field of lymphocytic colitis. Although challenges exist, the scientific community is increasingly recognizing the importance of studying this condition, and significant progress has been made in recent years.

As research continues to advance, the future holds promise for more personalized treatment options, a better understanding of the condition's causes, and enhanced support for individuals living with lymphocytic colitis. Advocacy and awareness efforts will play a crucial role in driving research and improving the lives of those affected by this condition.

Through ongoing collaboration between researchers, healthcare providers, patients, and advocacy groups, we can look forward to a brighter future for lymphocytic colitis, where effective treatments and support are more readily available, and individuals with the condition can lead fulfilling lives.

CHAPTER 8

Empowering Patients and Conclusion

In this final chapter, we will focus on empowering individuals living with lymphocytic colitis and provide a comprehensive conclusion to our exploration of this condition. Empowerment means equipping patients with the knowledge, resources, and support they need to take an active role in managing their health and improving their quality of life.

Patient-Centered Care

Empowering individuals with lymphocytic colitis begins with a patient-centered approach to care. This approach recognizes that each patient is unique, and their experiences and needs should guide their medical journey. Here are key components of patient-centered care:

1. **Shared Decision-Making:** Healthcare providers should engage patients in discussions about their treatment options, allowing them to make informed decisions that

align with their values and
preferences.

2. **Education:** Patients should
   receive clear and
   comprehensive information
   about their condition,
   treatment options, and
   lifestyle recommendations.
   Understanding empowers
   individuals to actively
   participate in their care.

3. **Access to Resources:**
   Patients should have access
   to resources and support
   networks, including
   advocacy groups, where they
   can find information, share
   experiences, and connect

with others facing similar challenges.

4. **Open Communication:** Effective communication between patients and healthcare providers is vital. Patients should feel comfortable asking questions, expressing concerns, and discussing their symptoms and treatment goals.

Self-Advocacy and Communication

Effective self-advocacy is a critical skill for individuals living with lymphocytic colitis. Here are some key principles to keep in mind:

1. **Know Your Condition:** Educate yourself about lymphocytic colitis, its symptoms, and treatment options. Understanding your condition empowers you to ask informed questions and make decisions about your care.

2. **Communication:** Be open and honest with your healthcare provider about your symptoms, treatment preferences, and concerns. Effective communication is

key to receiving the best care possible.

3. **Ask Questions:** Don't hesitate to ask questions or seek clarification during medical appointments. It's your health, and you have the right to understand your treatment plan.

4. **Seek Second Opinions:** If you are unsure about your diagnosis or treatment plan, don't hesitate to seek a second opinion from another healthcare provider. It's a common practice in medicine, and it can provide valuable insights.

Lifestyle Empowerment

In addition to medical treatment, lifestyle plays a crucial role in managing lymphocytic colitis. Empowering individuals to make healthy lifestyle choices can have a significant impact on their well-being:

1. **Dietary Management:** Work with a registered dietitian to create a personalized diet plan that minimizes symptom triggers while providing essential nutrients. Keeping a food diary can help identify

specific foods that worsen symptoms.

2. **Hydration:** Stay well-hydrated to prevent dehydration, a common concern with chronic diarrhea. Sipping water throughout the day and considering oral rehydration solutions can help.

3. **Stress Management:** Incorporate stress-reduction techniques into your daily routine, such as meditation, deep breathing exercises, or yoga. Reducing stress can help minimize symptom exacerbation.

4. **Physical Activity:** Engage in regular physical activity, as it can promote overall well-being. Consult your healthcare provider before starting any new exercise program.

Support Networks

Support networks are invaluable for individuals living with lymphocytic colitis. These networks provide emotional support, share practical tips, and raise awareness about the condition. Here's how to tap into support networks:

1. **Online Communities:**
   Join online forums, social
   media groups, or dedicated
   websites where individuals
   with lymphocytic colitis
   share their experiences and
   insights.

2. **Patient Advocacy
   Groups:** Many advocacy
   groups focus on
   gastrointestinal conditions
   like lymphocytic colitis.
   These organizations offer
   resources, support, and
   opportunities to get involved
   in advocacy efforts.

3. **Peer Support:** Connect
   with individuals who have

experience living with lymphocytic colitis. Hearing their stories and learning from their journeys can be incredibly empowering.

The Power of Education

Education is a cornerstone of empowerment. Individuals with lymphocytic colitis should actively seek knowledge about their condition and treatment options. Here are some educational aspects to consider:

1. **Stay Informed:** Keep up-to-date with the latest research and developments

related to lymphocytic colitis. Knowledge is a powerful tool in managing your health.

2. **Educate Others:** Share information about lymphocytic colitis with your friends and family. Increasing awareness can lead to better understanding and support from your loved ones.

3. **Advocate for Yourself:** Advocate for your needs within the healthcare system. If you encounter challenges or feel that your concerns are not being

addressed, don't hesitate to
speak up and seek solutions.

CONCLUSION

In this book, we've embarked on a journey to explore lymphocytic colitis comprehensively. We've covered its definition, symptoms, diagnosis, potential causes, treatment options, and research advancements. Most importantly, we've focused on the empowerment of individuals living with lymphocytic colitis.

Living with a chronic condition like lymphocytic colitis can be challenging, but it's essential to remember that you are not alone. Many resources and support networks are available to help you navigate this journey. By taking an active role in your care, advocating for your needs, and seeking support, you can improve your quality of life and face the challenges of lymphocytic colitis with resilience and determination.

As we conclude this book, we encourage you to continue your journey of empowerment. Stay informed, connect with others, and work closely with your healthcare provider to manage your condition effectively. Your health and well-being are worth the effort, and there is hope for a brighter and more empowered future in your journey with lymphocytic colitis.

In conclusion, our exploration of lymphocytic colitis has provided a comprehensive understanding of this chronic gastrointestinal condition. We've delved into its definition, symptoms, diagnosis, potential causes, treatment options, research advancements, and strategies for empowerment. Throughout this journey, we've emphasized the importance of patient-centered care, self-advocacy, and the power of education and support networks.

Living with lymphocytic colitis can present challenges, from the daily management of symptoms to the emotional impact it may have on individuals and their families. However, it's crucial to recognize that there is hope and a path toward a better quality of life.

Empowerment is at the heart of managing lymphocytic colitis. Empowered individuals are informed, actively involved in their healthcare decisions, and connected to support networks that provide understanding and encouragement. They are resilient in the face of challenges and are committed to improving their well-being.

As our understanding of lymphocytic colitis continues to evolve through ongoing research, advancements in personalized medicine, and increased awareness, the future holds promise for better treatments and improved support for those affected by this condition.

In your journey with lymphocytic colitis, remember that you are not alone. Support is available, and many individuals and organizations are dedicated to raising awareness and advocating for those living with this condition.

We hope this book has been a valuable resource in your quest for knowledge and empowerment. As you move forward, continue to seek information, communicate openly with your healthcare provider, and connect with others who share your experiences. Your health and well-being are worth the effort, and there is a community of support ready to stand with you on your journey with lymphocytic colitis.